Common Modifiers

Modifier 76 - Repeat Procedure or Service by the Same Physician or Other Qualified Health Care Professional:
- Used when a procedure or service is repeated by the same physician or provider.

MODIFIER 77 - REPEAT PROCEDURE BY ANOTHER PHYSICIAN:
- Indicates that a procedure or service was repeated by another provider after the original service.

Modifier 78 - Unplanned Return to the Operating/Procedure Room by the Same Physician Following Initial Procedure for a Related Procedure During the Postoperative Period:
- Used when a patient returns to the operating room for a related but unplanned procedure during the postoperative period of the initial surgery.

Modifier 79 - Unrelated Procedure or Service by the Same Physician During the Postoperative Period:
- Used when a procedure or service performed during the postoperative period was unrelated to the original procedure.

MODIFIER 80 - ASSISTANT SURGEON:
- Used when a second surgeon provides assistance during a surgical procedure.

MODIFIER 81 - MINIMUM ASSISTANT SURGEON:
- Indicates that a second surgeon provided minimal assistance during a surgical procedure.

Modifier 82 - Assistant Surgeon (When Qualified Resident Surgeon Not Available):
- Used when an assistant surgeon is required due to the unavailability of a qualified resident.

Modifier 91 - Repeat Clinical Diagnostic Laboratory Test:
- Indicates that the same laboratory test was performed multiple times on the same day for the same patient.

Modifier 90 - Reference (Outside) Laboratory:
- Indicates that laboratory procedures were performed by a party other than the treating or reporting physician.

Modifier 92 – Alternative Laboratory Platform Testing:
- Indicates testing performed using a kit or transportable instrument that requires a single-use, disposable analytical chamber.

Modifier 95 - Synchronous Telemedicine Service Rendered via a Real-Time Interactive Audio and Video Telecommunications System:
- Used to indicate services provided via telehealth where the provider and patient interact in real-time.

geniusgurulearning.org

Common Modifiers

Modifier 97 – Rehabilitative Services:
• Identifies rehabilitative services, which are services that help a person regain skills or functioning after illness or injury.

Modifier 99 – Multiple Modifiers:
• Used when multiple modifiers are necessary to fully describe a service.

Modifier 96 - Habilitative Services:
• Identifies habilitative services, which are services that help a person keep, learn, or improve skills and functioning for daily living.

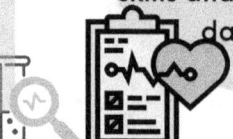

Modifier 99: Reference (Outside) Laboratory:
• Indicates that laboratory procedures were performed by a party other than the treating or reporting physician.

Modifiers means.....

Billing coding modifiers are used in medical billing to provide additional information about the performed procedure, service, or supply. They help specify the circumstances under which a procedure was performed without changing the overall definition of the code itself. Modifiers are essential for accurate billing and reimbursement processes, as they provide details that can affect payment.

geniusgurulearning.org

Common Modifiers

Modifier 22 - Increased Procedural Services:
- Indicates that the work required to perform a service was substantially greater than typically required.

Modifier 23 - Unusual Anesthesia:
- Used when general anesthesia is administered for a procedure that usually requires either no anesthesia or local anesthesia.

MODIFIER 25
SIGNIFICANT, SEPARATELY IDENTIFIABLE EVALUATION AND MANAGEMENT SERVICE BY THE SAME PHYSICIAN ON THE SAME DAY OF THE PROCEDURE OR OTHER SERVICE:
Used to indicate that a significant, separately identifiable evaluation and management (E/M) service was performed by the same physician on the same day as another procedure.

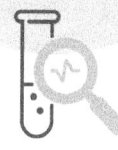

Modifier 26 - Professional Component:
- Used to indicate that a physician provided only the professional component of a service, such as interpreting an x-ray or ECG.

Modifier 27 - Multiple Outpatient Hospital E/M Encounters on the Same Date:
- Used to report multiple outpatient hospital Evaluation and Management (E/M) encounters performed on the same date.

Modifier 33 - Preventive Services:
- Used to identify preventive services. This modifier is often used for services where patient cost-sharing does not apply under applicable law.

Modifier 47 - Anesthesia by Surgeon:
- Used to indicate that the surgeon provided regional or general anesthesia for the surgical procedure.

Modifier 50 - Bilateral Procedure:
- Used to indicate that a bilateral procedure was performed, meaning the same procedure was performed on both sides of the body.

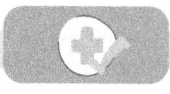

Modifier 51 - Multiple Procedures:
- Used when multiple procedures are performed during the same surgical session. This modifier informs the payer to reduce the payment for the secondary and subsequent procedures, as they often take less time compared to the first procedure.

Modifier 52 - Reduced Services:
- Used when a service or procedure is partially reduced or eliminated at the physician's discretion.

Modifier 54 - Surgical Care Only:
- Used when a provider performs only the surgical portion of a procedure and not the pre- or post-operative management.

geniusgurulearning.org

Common Modifiers

MODIFIER LT/RT - LEFT SIDE/RIGHT SIDE:
- Used to specify the side of the body where the procedure was performed (LT for left, RT for right).

MODIFIER 55 - POSTOPERATIVE MANAGEMENT ONLY:
INDICATES THAT THE PROVIDER RENDERED ONLY THE POSTOPERATIVE CARE

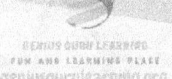

Modifier 56 - Preoperative Management Only:
- Used when a provider performs only the preoperative care and not the surgery or postoperative care.

Modifier 57 - Decision for Surgery:
- Used to indicate that an E/M service resulted in the initial decision to perform surgery.

Modifier 58 - Staged or Related Procedure or Service by the Same Physician During the Postoperative Period:
- Indicates a planned or staged procedure during the postoperative period of the initial surgery.

Modifier 62 - Two Surgeons:
- Indicates that two surgeons worked together as primary surgeons, each performing distinct parts of a procedure.

Modifier 63 - Procedure Performed on Infants Less than 4 kg:
- Used to indicate procedures performed on infants weighing less than 4 kilograms.

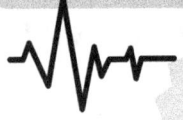
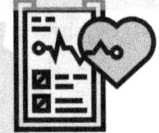
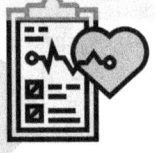
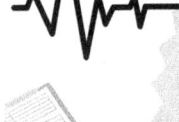

Modifier 59 – Distinct Procedural Service:
- Indicates that a procedure or service was distinct or independent from other services performed on the same day. It's often used to prevent bundling of services that should be paid separately.

Modifier 74 - Discontinued Outpatient Hospital/Ambulatory Surgery Center (ASC) Procedure After Administration of Anesthesia:
- Indicates a procedure was discontinued after anesthesia was administered.

MODIFIER 66 - SURGICAL TEAM:
- Used when a complex procedure requires the services of several surgeons, often of different specialties, working together as a team.

Modifier 73 - Discontinued Outpatient Hospital/Ambulatory Surgery Center (ASC) Procedure Prior to the Administration of Anesthesia:
- Indicates a procedure was discontinued after the patient was prepared for surgery but before anesthesia was administered.

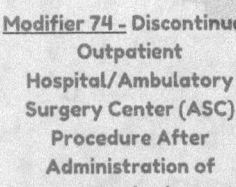

Common Modifiers

Modifier CA – Procedure payable only in the inpatient setting when performed emergently on an outpatient who dies prior to admission:
- Indicates that the procedure is typically performed inpatient, but was done emergently on an outpatient who subsequently died.

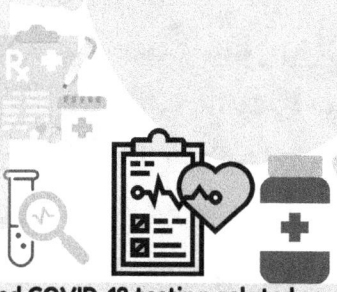

Modifier CS – Cost-sharing for specified COVID-19 testing-related services that result in an order for or administration of a COVID-19 test:
- Used during the COVID-19 pandemic to indicate services related to testing for COVID-19, for which cost-sharing is waived.

Modifier GC – This service has been performed in part by a resident under the direction of a teaching physician:
- Used to indicate that a resident provided part of the service under the supervision of a teaching physician.

Modifier GE - This service has been performed by a resident without the presence of a teaching physician under the primary care exception:
- Used for services provided by a resident without the direct supervision of a teaching physician under certain primary care exception rules.

9. Modifier GY – Item or service statutorily excluded or does not meet the definition of any Medicare benefit:
- Indicates that the item or service is excluded from Medicare coverage or does not meet the definition of a covered service.

Modifier GZ – Item or service expected to be denied as not reasonable and necessary:
- Used when an item or service is expected to be denied due to being not reasonable and necessary, and no Advanced Beneficiary Notice (ABN) was obtained.

Modifier KX – Requirements specified in the medical policy have been met:
- Indicates that the provider attests that the requirements of a medical policy have been met.

Modifier Q5 – Service furnished by a substitute physician under a reciprocal billing arrangement:
- Used to indicate services provided by a substitute physician under a reciprocal billing arrangement.

Modifier P1-P6 – Physical Status Modifiers (Anesthesia):
- These modifiers indicate the physical status of a patient undergoing anesthesia.
- P1: A normal healthy patient.
- P2: A patient with mild systemic disease.
- P3: A patient with severe systemic disease.
- P4: A patient with severe systemic disease that is a constant threat to life.
- P5: A moribund patient who is not expected to survive without the operation.
- P6: A declared brain-dead patient whose organs are being removed for donor purposes.

geniusgurulearning.org

Modifiers for Laboratory Services

Modifier Q6 - Service furnished by a locum tenens physician:
- Indicates services provided by a locum tenens (substitute) physician.

Modifier QJ - Services/items provided to a prisoner or patient in state or local custody:
- Used to indicate that services or items were provided to a patient who is incarcerated or in the custody of law enforcement.

Modifier QW - CLIA Waived Test:
- Indicates that the test performed is CLIA-waived (requires minimal oversight).

Modifiers for Imaging Services:

- **Modifier TC - Technical Component:**
- Indicates that only the technical component of a service, such as the equipment and technician services, was provided.
- **Modifier PC - Professional Component:**
- Indicates that only the professional component, such as the interpretation by a physician, was provided.

Modifier T1–T9 – Toe Modifiers:
- Used to specify which toe is involved in a procedure or service.
  - T1: Left foot, second digit.
  - T2: Left foot, third digit.
  - T3: Left foot, fourth digit.
  - T4: Left foot, fifth digit.
  - T5: Right foot, great toe.
  - T6: Right foot, second digit.
  - T7: Right foot, third digit.
  - T8: Right foot, fourth digit.
  - T9: Right foot, fifth digit.

Modifier for Use in ER Services:

- Modifier 27 - Multiple Outpatient Hospital E/M Encounters on the Same Date:
- Used to report multiple E/M services provided on the same date by the same or different providers in the same hospital setting.

Modifier G8 - Monitored anesthesia care (MAC) for deep complex, complicated, or markedly invasive surgical procedures:
- Indicates the provision of monitored anesthesia care (MAC) for more complex procedures.

geniusgurulearning.org

Modifiers for Laboratory Services

Modifier G9 - Monitored anesthesia care (MAC) for patient with history of severe cardiopulmonary condition:
- Indicates the use of MAC for a patient with a significant cardiopulmonary history.

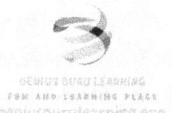

Modifier RA – Replacement of a DME item:
- Indicates replacement of a durable medical equipment item.

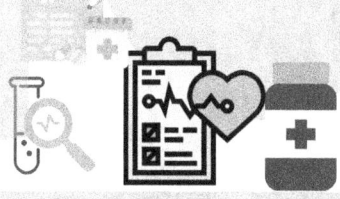

Modifier EP - Service provided as part of Medicaid Early and Periodic Screening, Diagnosis, and Treatment (EPSDT) program:
- Indicates services provided as part of the EPSDT program.

Modifier ET – Emergency Services:
- Used to denote services provided in an emergency situation.

Modifier FX - X-ray taken using film:
- Indicates that an X-ray was taken using film, rather than digital technology.

Modifier QJ – Services/items provided to a prisoner or patient in state or local custody:
- Used to indicate that services or items were provided to a patient who is incarcerated or in the custody of law enforcement.

Modifier GO – Telehealth services for diagnosis, evaluation, or treatment of symptoms of an acute stroke:
- Used for telehealth services provided for acute stroke evaluation.

Modifier RB – Replacement of a part of DME furnished as part of a repair:
- Indicates replacement of a component of durable medical equipment as part of a repair.

geniusgurulearning.org

Modifiers for Laboratory Services

Modifiers for Assistant at Surgery:

- **Modifier AS** - Physician Assistant, Nurse Practitioner, or Clinical Nurse Specialist Services for Assistant at Surgery:
  - Used to indicate that a physician assistant, nurse practitioner, or clinical nurse specialist is acting as an assistant at surgery.

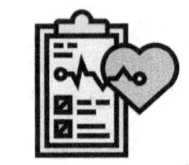

Modifiers for Audiology Services:

- **Modifier AU** - Item furnished in conjunction with a hearing aid:
  - Indicates items provided in conjunction with a hearing aid.
- **Modifier AV** - Item furnished in conjunction with a cochlear implant:
  - Indicates items provided in conjunction with a cochlear implant.
- **Modifier AW** - Item furnished in conjunction with a wheelchair:
  - Indicates items provided in conjunction with a wheelchair.

Modifiers for Mental Health Services:

- Modifier AH - Clinical Psychologist
- Modifier AJ - Clinical Social Worker
- Modifier HO - Master's Level
- Modifier HP - Doctoral Level
- Modifier HN - Bachelor's Level

Modifiers for Fingers:

- **Modifier F1** - Left hand, second digit (index finger)
- **Modifier F2** - Left hand, third digit (middle finger)
- **Modifier F3** - Left hand, fourth digit (ring finger)
- **Modifier F4** - Left hand, fifth digit (little finger)
- **Modifier F5** - Right hand, thumb
- **Modifier F6** - Right hand, second digit (index finger)
- **Modifier F7** - Right hand, third digit (middle finger)
- **Modifier F8** - Right hand, fourth digit (ring finger)
- **Modifier F9** - Right hand, fifth digit (little finger)

MODIFIERS FOR AMBULANCE SERVICES:

- **Modifier GM** - Multiple patients on one ambulance trip
- **Modifier QL** - Patient pronounced dead after ambulance called

MODIFIERS FOR EYES:

- **Modifier E1** - Upper left eyelid
- **Modifier E2** - Lower left eyelid
- **Modifier E3** - Upper right eyelid
- **Modifier E4** - Lower right eyelid

geniusgurulearning.org

Miscellaneous Modifiers:

- **Modifier XU** - Unusual Non-Overlapping Service, the use of a service that is distinct because it does not overlap usual components of the main service
- **Modifier XP** - Separate Practitioner, a service that is distinct because it was performed by a different practitioner
- **Modifier XS** - Separate Structure, a service that is distinct because it was performed on a separate organ/structure
- **Modifier XE** - Separate Encounter, a service that is distinct because it occurred during a separate encounter

Modifiers for Services Provided by Physician Extenders:

- **Modifier SA** - Nurse Practitioner rendering service in collaboration with a physician
- **Modifier SB** - Nurse midwife
- **Modifier U1-U9** - State specific use only

Modifiers for Certified Registered Nurse Anesthetist (CRNA):

- **Modifier QX** - CRNA service with medical direction by a physician
- **Modifier QZ** - CRNA service without medical direction by a physician

MODIFIERS FOR LABORATORY SERVICES:

- **Modifier 32** - Mandated Services: Used to identify services that are required by a third party, such as a government, court order, or insurance carrier
- **Modifier 90** - Reference (Outside) Laboratory

Modifiers for Pediatric Services:

- **Modifier HA** - Child/adolescent program
- **Modifier HB** - Adult program, non-geriatric
- **Modifier HC** - Senior citizen program, geriatric

Modifiers for Services in Teaching Settings:

- **Modifier GC** - This service has been performed in part by a resident under the direction of a teaching physician
- **Modifier GE** - This service has been performed by a resident without the presence of a teaching physician under the primary care exception

Modifiers for Right and Left Sides of the Body:

- **Modifier RT** - Right Side (used to identify procedures performed on the right side of the body)
- **Modifier LT** - Left Side (used to identify procedures performed on the left side of the body)

geniusgurulearning.org

Anesthesia Modifiers:

- AA – Anesthesia services performed personally by the anesthesiologist
- QK – Medical direction of two, three, or four concurrent anesthesia procedures involving qualified individuals
- QX – CRNA service with medical direction by a physician
- QY – Medical direction of one CRNA by an anesthesiologist
- QZ – CRNA service without medical direction by a physician

Category II Modifiers (Performance Measures)

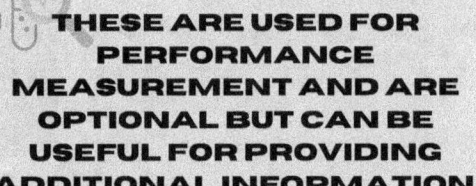

THESE ARE USED FOR PERFORMANCE MEASUREMENT AND ARE OPTIONAL BUT CAN BE USEFUL FOR PROVIDING ADDITIONAL INFORMATION.

- 1P – Performance Measure Exclusion Modifier Due to Medical Reasons
- 2P – Performance Measure Exclusion Modifier Due to Patient Choice
- 3P – Performance Measure Exclusion Modifier Due to System Reasons
- 8P – Performance Measure Reporting Modifier (Action Not Performed, Reason Not Otherwise Specified)

Modifiers for Global Surgery Periods:

- 24 - Unrelated Evaluation and Management Service by the Same Physician During a Postoperative Period
- 25 - Significant, Separately Identifiable Evaluation and Management Service by the Same Physician on the Same Day of the Procedure or Other Service
- 57 - Decision for Surgery
- 58 - Staged or Related Procedure or Service by the Same Physician During the Postoperative Period
- 78 - Unplanned Return to the Operating/Procedure Room by the Same Physician Following Initial Procedure for a Related Procedure During the Postoperative Period
- 79 - Unrelated Procedure or Service by the Same Physician During the Postoperative Period

geniusgurulearning.org

	Common Modifiers	
22	Increased procedural services	Complex surgeries requiring extra time and effort
24	Unrelated evaluation and management service by the same physician during a postoperative period	Follow-up office visit for a condition not related to the surgery
25	Significant, separately identifiable evaluation and management service by the same physician on the same day of the procedure or other service	Patient with multiple concerns addressed during a single visit
26	Professional component	Radiologist interpretation of an X-ray
32	Mandated services	Services required by a third party, like a government agency
50	Bilateral procedure	Knee surgery performed on both knees
51	Multiple procedures	Removal of a mole and a wart during the same visit
52	Reduced services	Partial removal of a lesion
53	Discontinued procedure	Stopping a colonoscopy due to complications
54	Surgical care only	Surgeon performs only the operation, not the aftercare
55	Postoperative management only	Postoperative care after surgery is managed by a different provider
56	Preoperative management only	Preoperative visit only, not including the surgery itself
57	Decision for surgery	Consultation leading to surgery
58	Staged or related procedure or service by the same physician during the postoperative period	Second procedure related to the first, during the recovery period

	Common Modifiers	
59	Distinct procedural service	Separate diagnostic procedure performed during surgery
62	Two surgeons	Two surgeons working together on a complex surgery
63	Procedure performed on infants less than 4 kg	Surgery on a premature infant weighing less than 4 kg
76	Repeat procedure or service by the same physician or other qualified health care professional	Repeat blood test by the same doctor on the same day
77	Repeat procedure by another physician or other qualified health care professional	Repeat X-ray by another doctor
78	Unplanned return to the operating/procedure room by the same physician following initial procedure for a related procedure during the postoperative period	Second surgery due to complications from the first
79	Unrelated procedure or service by the same physician during the postoperative period	Unrelated surgery during the recovery period of another surgery
80	Assistant surgeon	A surgical assistant is present during the surgery
81	Minimum assistant surgeon	Resident in training assists during the surgery
82	Assistant surgeon (when qualified resident surgeon not available)	Emergency surgery where no resident was available
AS	Physician assistant, nurse practitioner, or clinical nurse specialist services for assistant at surgery	Nurse practitioner assists in surgery
E1	Upper left eyelid	Excision of a lesion on the upper left eyelid
E2	Lower left eyelid	Removal of a cyst on the lower left eyelid
E3	Upper right eyelid	Biopsy of a lesion on the upper right eyelid

	Common Modifiers	
E4	Lower right eyelid	Biopsy of a lesion on the upper right eyelid
F1	Left hand, second digit	Excision of a growth on the lower right eyelid
F2	Left hand, third digit	Fracture repair on the left index finger
F3	Left hand, fourth digit	Removal of a wart on the left middle finger
F4	Left hand, fifth digit	Nail repair on the left ring finger
F5	Right hand, thumb	Skin biopsy on the left little finger
F6	Right hand, second digit	Suture of a laceration on the right thumb
F7	Right hand, third digit	Wound care on the right index finger
F8	Right hand, fourth digit	Fracture reduction on the right middle finger
F9	Right hand, fifth digit	Nail removal on the right ring finger
GA	Waiver of liability statement issued as required by payer policy, individual case	Infection treatment on the right little finger
GC	This service has been performed in part by a resident under the direction of a teaching physician	Notice given to the patient that the service may not be covered
GE	This service has been performed by a resident without the presence of a teaching physician under the primary care exception	Part of a procedure performed by a resident under supervision

Common Modifiers

GG	PERFORMANCE AND PAYMENT OF A SCREENING MAMMOGRAM AND DIAGNOSTIC MAMMOGRAM ON THE SAME PATIENT, SAME DAY	SCREENING MAMMOGRAM FOLLOWED BY A DIAGNOSTIC MAMMOGRAM
GQ	VIA ASYNCHRONOUS TELECOMMUNICATIONS SYSTEM	TELEHEALTH CONSULTATION VIA STORE-AND-FORWARD TECHNOLOGY
GT	VIA INTERACTIVE AUDIO AND VIDEO TELECOMMUNICATION SYSTEMS	REAL-TIME TELEHEALTH CONSULTATION
GZ	ITEM OR SERVICE EXPECTED TO BE DENIED AS NOT REASONABLE AND NECESSARY	ITEM PROVIDED EVEN THOUGH IT IS EXPECTED TO BE DENIED BY INSURANCE
KX	REQUIREMENTS SPECIFIED IN THE MEDICAL POLICY HAVE BEEN MET	INDICATION THAT SPECIFIC MEDICAL POLICY REQUIREMENTS WERE MET
LT	LEFT SIDE	SURGERY PERFORMED ON THE LEFT KNEE
RT	RIGHT SIDE	SURGERY PERFORMED ON THE RIGHT SHOULDER
QX	CRNA SERVICE WITH MEDICAL DIRECTION BY A PHYSICIAN	CRNA PROVIDES ANESTHESIA WITH OVERSIGHT FROM A PHYSICIAN
QZ		CRNA PROVIDES ANESTHESIA WITHOUT OVERSIGHT FROM A PHYSICIAN
TI	LEFT FOOT, SECOND DIGIT	INGROWN TOENAIL REMOVAL ON THE LEFT SECOND TOE

Common Modifiers

T2	Left foot, third digit	Wart removal on the left third toe
T3	Left foot, fourth digit	Fracture care on the left fourth toe
T4	Left foot, fifth digit	Toenail removal on the left fifth toe
T5	Right foot, great toe	Bunionectomy on the right big toe
T6	Right foot, second digit	Surgical repair of a fracture on the right second toe
T7	Right foot, third digit	Wound care on the right third toe
T8	Right foot, fourth digit	Corn removal on the right fourth toe
T9	Right foot, fifth digit	Toenail trimming on the right fifth toe
XE	Separate Encounter, A Service That Is Distinct Because It Occurred During A Separate Encounter	Separate office visit on the same day for a different problem
XP	Separate Practitioner, A Service That Is Distinct Because It Was Performed By A Different Practitioner	Same procedure performed by a different doctor
XS	Separate Structure, A Service That Is Distinct Because It Was Performed On A Separate Organ/Structure	Procedure performed on a separate anatomical site
XU	Unusual Non-Overlapping Service, The Use Of A Service That Is Distinct Because It Does Not Overlap Usual Components Of The Main Service	Service that doesn't overlap with the main procedure

Medical billing professionals play a crucial role in the healthcare industry by ensuring that medical services are accurately billed and that insurance claims are processed efficiently. There are several types of medical billing professionals, each with distinct roles and responsibilities. Here's a breakdown of the main types:

1. Medical Billers

Role: Medical billers are responsible for preparing and submitting claims to insurance companies. They review patient records, code diagnoses and procedures, and ensure that claims are complete and accurate.

Key Responsibilities:
Coding medical procedures and diagnoses.
Submitting claims to insurance companies.
Follow-up on denied claims and appeals.
Verifying patient information and insurance coverage.

2. Medical Coders

Role: Medical coders convert healthcare diagnoses, procedures, and services into standardized codes. These codes are used for billing purposes and to ensure accurate and consistent medical records.

Key Responsibilities:
Assigning codes to medical diagnoses and procedures based on medical records.
Ensuring codes are accurate and up-to-date with current coding systems (ICD-10, CPT, HCPCS).
Collaborating with medical billers to ensure accurate billing.

3. Medical Billing and Coding Specialists

Role: These professionals handle both billing and coding tasks. They are versatile and capable of managing both the coding of medical services and the submission of insurance claims.

Key Responsibilities:
Combining responsibilities of both medical billers and coders.
Handling the full spectrum of billing and coding tasks.
Ensuring compliance with healthcare regulations and insurance policies.

4. Claims Examiners

Role: Claims examiners review insurance claims to determine their validity and ensure they meet the insurer's criteria. They work for insurance companies to manage and process claims.

Key Responsibilities:
Reviewing and verifying claims submitted by medical billers.
Determining if claims meet policy terms and conditions.
Investigating and resolving discrepancies or issues with claims.

5. Medical Billing Managers

Role: Medical billing managers oversee billing departments or teams. They ensure that billing processes are efficient and compliant with regulations.

Key Responsibilities:
Supervising medical billers and coders.
Developing and implementing billing procedures.
Managing billing software and systems.
Handling complex billing issues and insurance disputes.

6. Medical Reimbursement Specialists

Role: These specialists focus on the reimbursement process, ensuring that healthcare providers receive payment for services rendered.

Key Responsibilities:
Reviewing and processing reimbursements.
Managing payer contracts and reimbursement rates.
Addressing issues related to underpayments or delays in payments.

Key Differences:
Scope of Work: Medical billers focus primarily on the submission and management of claims, while coders focus on accurately coding medical information. Specialists in both roles handle a broader range of tasks, including both billing and coding.
Work Environment: Billers and coders may work in healthcare facilities, insurance companies, or from home. Managers and examiners often work within insurance companies or large healthcare organizations.
Training and Certification: The qualifications can vary; billers and coders often require specific training and certifications (e.g., Certified Professional Coder, Certified Billing and Coding Specialist). Managers and examiners may need additional experience and skills in leadership and claims processing.
Each type of medical billing professional plays a vital role in ensuring the smooth operation of healthcare financial processes, ultimately contributing to the overall efficiency and accuracy of healthcare administration.

Here's a breakdown of Level 3 codes across various coding systems:

1. CPT Level 3 Codes

Level 3 codes in the Current Procedural Terminology (CPT) system were formerly used to describe office or other outpatient consultations and other services. However, these codes have been largely replaced or reclassified. For example: 99341-99350 were used for home or office visits, but with changes in coding guidelines and updates to the CPT codes, many of these have been replaced or modified.

2. HCPCS Level 3 Codes

HCPCS Level 3 codes (also known as Local Codes) were used to provide additional codes for services and equipment not covered by Level 1 (CPT) or Level 2 codes. These codes were used by Medicare contractors to identify specific services or supplies in particular regions. However, HCPCS Level 3 codes have been discontinued and are no longer in use. They have been replaced by:
HCPCS Level 1 codes (CPT codes)
HCPCS Level 2 codes (for non-physician services like durable medical equipment, prosthetics, orthotics, and supplies)

3. ICD-10-CM Codes

In the ICD-10-CM (International Classification of Diseases, 10th Revision, Clinical Modification) system, there isn't a Level 3 coding designation. Instead, ICD-10-CM uses a more detailed structure with codes that can go up to 7 characters. The structure includes:

3-character codes for basic categories.

4-7 character codes to provide more detail and specificity.

4. Coding Levels in Practice Management

In some practice management or coding training contexts, coding levels might refer to the complexity of medical services and documentation required, such as:

Level 1: Basic, straightforward services.

Level 2: Moderate complexity services.

Level 3: High complexity services.

Level 4: Very high complexity services.

These levels often help in determining the complexity and time required for a service, impacting the billing and reimbursement process.

In Summary:

CPT Level 3 codes have been mostly phased out or reclassified.

HCPCS Level 3 codes are no longer in use; replaced by Levels 1 and 2.

ICD-10-CM does not have a Level 3 designation but uses a multi-character coding structure.

Coding levels in practice management may denote service complexity.

Understanding these coding systems and their updates is crucial for accurate medical billing and compliance. For up-to-date information, always refer to the latest coding manuals and guidelines.

Below is a summary of various medical coding systems and the meanings of some commonly used codes within each system. This should provide a good overview of how codes are used in different contexts:

1. CPT (Current Procedural Terminology) Codes

Purpose: CPT codes are used to describe medical, surgical, and diagnostic services and procedures.

99213: Established Patient Office Visit, Moderate Complexity - A visit with an established patient, typically requiring 15-30 minutes of face-to-face time with the patient.

20610: Arthrocentesis, Aspiration, or Injection of Major Joint or Bursa - A procedure to remove fluid from or inject medication into a major joint.

99396: Periodic Comprehensive Preventive Medicine Evaluation and Management - A preventive exam for established patients, typically involving a thorough assessment and preventive services.

2. ICD-10-CM (International Classification of Diseases, 10th Revision, Clinical Modification) Codes

Purpose: ICD-10-CM codes are used to classify and code diagnoses, symptoms, and procedures.

E11.9: Type 2 Diabetes Mellitus without Complications - A diagnosis code for Type 2 diabetes without complications.

I10: Essential Hypertension - A diagnosis code for high blood pressure without a specified cause.

M54.5: Low Back Pain - A diagnosis code for pain located in the lower back.

3. HCPCS Level 2 Codes

Purpose: HCPCS Level 2 codes are used for billing non-physician services and supplies not covered by CPT codes.

A9270: Non-covered Item or Service - A code used to indicate that the item or service is not covered by the payer.

E0110: Crutches, Underarm, Wood or Aluminum, Each - A code for billing underarm crutches.

J codes (e.g., J2040): Injection, Erythropoietin, 1000 Units - Codes used for injectable drugs and biologicals.

4. CPT Modifiers

Purpose: Modifiers provide additional information about a service or procedure and may affect reimbursement.

25: Significant, Separately Identifiable Evaluation and Management Service - Used when a significant, separate evaluation and management service is provided on the same day as another procedure.

59: Distinct Procedural Service - Indicates that a procedure or service was distinct or independent from other services performed on the same day.

5. ICD-10-PCS (International Classification of Diseases, 10th Revision, Procedure Coding System) Codes

Purpose: ICD-10-PCS codes are used for inpatient procedure coding.

0DB98ZZ: Excision of the Left Ovary, Open Approach - A code for removing the left ovary through an open surgical approach.

2B1101Z: Insertion of a Synthetic Substitute into the Left Femur - A code for inserting a synthetic material into the left femur.

6. CPT Category II Codes

Purpose: CPT Category II codes are used for performance measurement and quality improvement.

3024F: Documentation of Tobacco Use Status - Used to indicate that the patient's tobacco use status has been documented.

3072F: Screening for Depression - Indicates that a depression screening was performed.

7. CPT Category III Codes

Purpose: CPT Category III codes are temporary codes for emerging technologies, services, and procedures.

0506T: Endoscopic Gastroplasty for Weight Reduction - A code for a new procedure related to weight reduction using endoscopic techniques.

These codes are essential for accurate documentation, billing, and insurance reimbursement in the healthcare industry. Each coding system serves a specific purpose, and proper usage ensures that healthcare services are appropriately classified and compensated

Studying medical coding and the associated costs can vary depending on the route you take. Here's a general overview:

Time Commitment

Formal Education: Many people opt for a formal education route, such as a certificate or associate degree program. These typically take about 6 months to 2 years to complete.

Self-Study: If you're studying independently or through online courses, the time can vary widely depending on your pace. It might take anywhere from a few months to over a year.

Certification Preparation: Preparing for certification exams (like the CPC from the AAPC or the CCS from the AHIMA) can add additional time, often a few months of focused study.

Costs

Educational Programs:

Certificate Programs: Usually cost between $1,000 and $3,000.

Associate Degree Programs: These can range from $5,000 to $15,000, depending on the institution.

Certification Exam Fees:

CPC (Certified Professional Coder): Approximately $300 to $400.

CCS (Certified Coding Specialist): Around $300 to $400.

Additional Costs:

Study Materials and Books: Around $100 to $300.

Membership Fees: Some professional organizations have membership fees, often ranging from $100 to $200 annually.

Other Considerations

Financial Aid: Some programs offer financial aid or payment plans.

Return on Investment: The cost of certification can often be offset by higher earning potential. Certified medical coders can earn a competitive salary, with the median annual wage in the U.S. often ranging between $50,000 and $60,000, depending on experience and location.

Planning your path and budget will help you manage the time and cost effectively.

www.ingramcontent.com/pod-product-compliance
Lightning Source LLC
Chambersburg PA
CBHW081022240526
45471CB00018B/3943